'When Emma turns her forensic gaze
on to a subject, that subject should be very
afraid. She is stepping out on to virgin
soil here and busting it open in the most
comprehensive of ways'
EMMA FREUD

'I can remember before I had a baby,
wondering and wondering what it would
feel like to be a mother and have a baby.
Maternity Service is a companion for mothers
and mothers-to-be who would like a bit of
realistic insight into what it might be like'
PHILIPPA PERRY, AUTHOR OF
*THE BOOK YOU WISH YOUR PARENTS
HAD READ (AND YOUR CHILDREN
WILL BE GLAD THAT YOU DID)*

Maternity Service

*A Love Letter to Mothers from the
Front Line of Maternity Leave*

EMMA BARNETT

FIG TREE
an imprint of
PENGUIN BOOKS

FIG TREE

UK | USA | Canada | Ireland | Australia
India | New Zealand | South Africa

Fig Tree is part of the Penguin Random House group of companies
whose addresses can be found at global.penguinrandomhouse.com

Penguin Random House UK,
One Embassy Gardens, 8 Viaduct Gardens, London SW11 7BW

penguin.co.uk

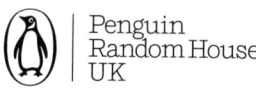

First published 2025

004

Set in 12.5/14.75pt Garamond MT Std
Typeset by Jouve (UK), Milton Keynes
Printed and bound in Great Britain by Clays Ltd, Elcograf S.p.A.

The authorized representative in the EEA is Penguin Random House Ireland,
Morrison Chambers, 32 Nassau Street, Dublin D02 YH68

A CIP catalogue record for this book is available from the British Library

ISBN: 978-0-241-69639-2

Penguin Random House is committed to a sustainable future
for our business, our readers and our planet. This book is made from
Forest Stewardship Council® certified paper.

Maternity Service

In one important sense maternity leave is poorly named, as it involves no actual leave. You are constantly on, even when your offspring is having a nap. There is nothing restful about it. In another sense, maternity leave is aptly named, because it's a period of leave from all you know: taking leave of one's mind, body, job and relationships.

When Emma Barnett began her second maternity leave, she realized that, despite having been there before, as soon as her first leave finished the rose-tinted lenses had descended and she immediately forgot what the experience was *actually* like when you're in it. This collective forgetting, which leads to well-meaning comments such as 'enjoy every minute' and 'treasure this special time', is doing a disservice to women, leaving them unprepared for the more complicated reality of what it means to be on maternity *service*.

In this warmly reassuring, refreshingly honest book, Emma sets out to capture this reality, in real time while on her latest tour of duty. She isn't offering advice on sleep-training or weaning or helping your baby reach milestones. Instead, this book is a celebration and acknowledgement of the *work* of being on maternity leave, with its soaring highs and challenging lows, and its impact on how women feel about our purpose and ourselves.

For my daughter, my girl.

Contents

CONTENTS

On Your Marks

Congratulations! You are a parent. A whole other person has joined your crew – and the rest of the human race – because of you. Welcome to this dazzling, emotional and utterly life-changing experience. Before you were one. Now you are two: divided – and connected – for evermore.

You will feel things you have never felt. You will do things you have never done. You will understand what it means to have one heart on the outside of your body while the original pumps madly to keep up with the new levels of love and anxiety coursing through you. Think falling in love with a partner was crazy and exhilarating? Try reproducing. You'll find yourself falling in love in a way you simply didn't know was possible.

You have done something incredible. As you have probably already found out, it ain't like the movies. Having a baby lifts the lid on a whole layer of life and existence you will have been oblivious to until now, despite having gone through it once before on the other side, as a babe in arms. Birth is wild. Never forget that. And you will need time to recover.

But once it's done, no matter what state it has left you in – it's done. And your new role begins immediately. This is where we meet each other. The starting blocks.

Before We Begin

I am writing this so I don't forget it because I know I will. We, as women, seem programmed to forget how maternity leave feels even as we experience it. Our memory just skips to the highlights reel and omits the other parts. I know, because I wiped the slate nearly clean after my last stint five years ago.

I am writing this because I think another woman will need to read it.

I am writing this because before my first maternity leave I hadn't considered how I might feel outside of my relationship to my baby during this time. I want to bear witness to those feelings, which I hope might resonate with some of your feelings too.

I am writing this because another older mother unintentionally made me feel bad for articulating some of these feelings.

I am writing this because despite the millions of words spilled about motherhood into books – I should know as I own at least fifteen of them – in none of them did I find what I am about to commit to paper in quite this way.

I am writing this as the single child of a mother who regularly proclaims that she adored every single minute of my existence, especially that first year, during which I apparently 'never really cried' and made for the most

joyful and fascinating company. While that total ador-
ation has bolstered my whole existence, as a new mother
who cannot claim the same experience, it's also provoked
many questions.

And finally I am writing this because I've just returned
home from an exercise class for new mothers who, despite looking a little like war veterans, splayed out awkwardly
on soft floor mats coping with a range of injuries, when
asked, largely said they were 'fine'.

So, when it was my turn to share my name, my six-
month-old daughter's name and how I was feeling, on an
extremely hot day sitting on the floor of a newly built
barn amongst the local community park greenhouses – I
felt it was my duty to say how I really was.

It went something like this: 'My name is Emma. This is
my daughter – whom I love very, very much. I have a hugely
painful herniated disc in my back, a hypertonic pelvic floor,
an ingrowing toenail which may now be infected, and I am
finding this pretty tough and mind-numbing.'

Slight intakes of breath all round – not least from the
smiling Zen teacher, who had clearly been hoping for
more positive energy. Although I also delivered it with a
big smile, which further confused matters. Then slowly,
but ever so surely, women around me broke into nervous
sweaty smiles and knowing nods.

Because, as I've alluded to, this maternity leave is not
my first rodeo. It's my second. Five years on. Our second
child, our daughter, miraculously appeared following six
rounds of IVF over three years – a soul-destroying,

mood-altering and incredibly draining experience I have written and talked publicly about.

If you are exceedingly lucky, IVF ends in maternity leave with a hopefully healthy baby.

But because it's my second maternity leave, I knew going into it that, rather ironically, despite the years of needles, drugs and tears I had endured to try and have a second child, this period of time would still not be the sweet, doting, fun-filled nirvana I had thought it might be the first time around. Instead, I understood that it would be filled with sweat, blood, milk, more tears and time. Vast oceans of the stuff.

So now I am trying to distil how this odd, precious and discombobulating time feels, before I forget it. Again.

The act of writing it has been more important to me than I could have imagined.

I hope it helps.

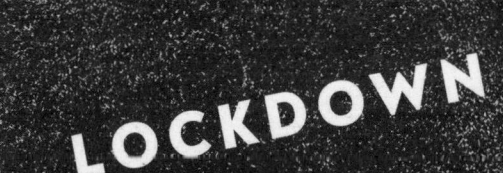

When the national Covid-19 lockdown happened in 2020, only two years after my first maternity leave with our son (whom I had also struggled to have after years of trying, a long overdue endometriosis diagnosis and IVF treatment), I remember thinking: uh oh – weeks at home, unable to leave the house easily, if at all, normal life suspended, with most hopes and dreams delayed for another day – I know this movie. I've seen a version of it before. It feels rather a lot like maternity leave.

Of course, the lockdown was far more serious, and the experience of it dramatically differed depending on your circumstances – not least if a loved one or yourself became unwell. Lives were lost, livelihoods destroyed, education severely interrupted and mental health issues ballooned as people were left isolated – chief amongst them new mothers. I was presenting the BBC 5 Live's mid-morning three-hour daily news programme during that time – some of it from my home – and it was extraordinary in the truest sense of the word, as I spoke to people in all types of situations and interviewed politicians across the country. At the same time I was also starting and then stopping IVF in an NHS hospital, largely on my own, as partners were no longer permitted at procedures or any health appointment.

But if you will humour me for a moment, lockdown

did present parallels with maternity leave, beyond loneliness and an immediate familiarity with every inch of one's local park. An existential crisis began for some of those who found themselves furloughed or suddenly working from home. Overnight, both men and women were left wondering who they were; what made them *them*? What was their purpose in life? Was this all life was? Were they living in the right place? And with the right people? Had they made the right choices, as time seemed to stand still? And all these questions were often being asked well before nine a.m. And then played on repeat throughout the day and the night.

Welcome to maternity leave, I thought with a wry smile – where you've seen the inside of a minute second by second, seen every hour of every day often from the same two positions in your house (from chair to bed and bed to chair). Although in lockdown you didn't necessarily also have to contend with having a newborn to care for, disrupting your every thought, just sitting or lying there being cute in a puddle of poo – still needing you to be on, but not *that* on. (I write this recognizing, of course, that some women's maternity leave collided with lockdown, which brought its own unique set of challenges. And I also know it sometimes led to amazing and unanticipated new experiences for people whose partners were suddenly, unexpectedly around and not working away from home.)

So here I am again. On mat leave. Three years after lockdown began and five years after my last time in the wilderness – because that is what maternity leave is. Whether you love or loathe it, or fall somewhere in between, it's properly and madly wild. An upside-down version of normal life, where everyone else still seems to be going on with their business and you are catapulted into a new space beneath, where you can see your old life but it is no longer within grasp. At least not for the foreseeable future.

I am also writing this in real time. In snatched moments while our daughter naps and our son is at school. I want to stress this because there is a deliberateness to the flurry of observations and the desperation to finish a train of thought, which I hope any woman on this road, past or present, can relate to. I have attempted to impose an order on it to help you map your way through, but there are times it spills over, because this clamour and over-bubbling is particularly unique to life with a very young baby and I don't want to hide that. It's central to what this book is about.

I want to embrace it as I share what I have learned. I want to paint a portrait and offer up some kind of map of the land I find myself in. Right now. In this moment. Before it has gone, before it has slipped through my fingers, and I am no longer on the front line of new motherhood. I know that on my first maternity leave – and, for that matter, at the start of this second one – I would have found it very useful to have been handed some sort of map, however sketchy, by another woman, reaching out to me through the sleep-deprived fog of love, hormones and utter confusion.

This is my attempt to send back dispatches from a level of life I hadn't known existed. And just like discovering a secret sub-world in a video game through a hidden door you hadn't realized was there until you pushed your way in, you'll find the rules are slightly different and everything seems somehow *off*, even though it might look familiar.

Hold that thought. If you can. It's time for some important caveats.

'NOT EVERY WOMAN'

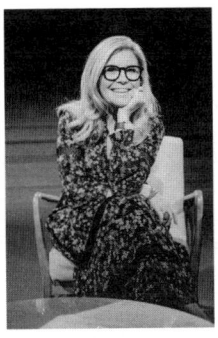

Emma Barnett is an award-winning broadcaster and journalist. She was named Interviewer of the Year for 2022 at the British Journalism awards and is a presenter on BBC Radio 4's flagship *Today* programme, as well as hosting TV interviews and documentaries across the BBC. She has presented programmes that include *Woman's Hour* on BBC Radio 4 and *Newsnight*. She also presented a global interviews programme on Bloomberg TV, interviewing international figures from across the world of politics, sport, entertainment and technology.

Emma pens a bi-weekly newspaper column for the *i*, and was previously a columnist for the *Sunday Times* and the *Daily Telegraph*, where she was also the Women's Editor. After the birth of her first child, she wrote *Period: It's about Bloody Time*, her first book.

Emma grew up in Manchester, and now lives in London with her husband and their two children.

I love my daughter with every fibre of my being. What I am about to write is not about her. In fact, I am writing it *because* of her and in a bid to be helpful to her – and other women – should she procreate at some point.

I know not everyone has maternity leave – even though technically it's a legal right. Not everyone can afford it, nor are they supported to do so.

I know not every woman wants to be on maternity leave for as long as they have to be but childcare costs are so prohibitive they end up staying as full-time carers for longer than they ever planned because they cannot afford to work.

I know some women want their maternity leave to be longer and cannot afford for that scenario to play out.

I know some women have no job to return to through no fault of their own due to maternity discrimination.

I know some women have zero family support or a decent friend network.

I know in some cases that the other parent is the main carer and the one who takes the most parental leave. I know some babies are not born well, and this whole time for their parents couldn't be further from what I am going to be writing about.

I know some babies rarely sleep or stop crying.

I know some women never get to this point despite throwing everything at it.

I know some women absolutely bloody love this time.

And finally, I know how lucky women in the UK and most of Europe are to have any period of leave, at least in principle, legally protected at twelve months, to be with their babies.

Despite the caveats above and the many more I have omitted, I would have felt a bit better on my first maternity leave if someone had shared this perspective with me. Because, weirdly, saying anything critical or even negative about maternity leave is often still frowned upon. Or it makes people rush to tell you that you might be depressed. Or that you just 'miss work'.

Luckily, I am not depressed, nor am I chomping at the bit to get back to my job – despite people constantly wanting to peg me solely as a 'career woman'. But what I do miss is me; a sense of self; a faster brain; a balance to my life.

This is not a book about the negatives and challenges of child-rearing. And how mundane it really is a lot of the time. Bloggers over the last two decades have blown the doors right off that one. The slummy mummy brigade is still going strong and all power to them. Although as a result it's now almost taboo to admit it if you actually like mothering and caring for young children.

Nor am I remotely qualified or in the market to give parenting tips to mothers. The concept of the 'good-enough mother' has been going strong since 1953 when it was coined by the British psychoanalyst and paediatrician

Donald Winnicott and picked up by feminist journalists such as Libby Purves with her book *How Not to Be a Perfect Mother*.

The philosophical, feminist and political side of what motherhood can do to women has also been wonderfully covered – increasingly so. We owe a debt to those who initially transgressed and sometimes paid a price for it. First mention goes to the important writing of Rachel Cusk, starting with her searing *A Life's Work*.

Julie Phillips's incredible book *The Baby on the Fire Escape: Creativity, Motherhood, and the Mind-Baby Problem* is one of the best books I have read about how to hold on to yourself while parenting, based on the lessons of others.

And, most recently, the essential *Matrescence* by the science journalist and good friend of mine Lucy Jones, explains how our brains, bodies and minds are changing as we go through a metamorphosis that must be acknowledged and catered for, just as we do for young people going through adolescence.

I also found Naomi Stadlen's book *What Mothers Do: especially when it looks like nothing* quietly ground-breaking on my first maternity leave as I struggled to get to grips with my new reality.

All of these I highly recommend to any woman as she starts on her road to motherhood.

But I also recommend this pithy and blisteringly honest quote from a producer who emailed me three months after I gave birth: 'I was bored and knackered and miserable for my mat leave with sparks of joy.'

I am also deliberately not focusing on the experiences

that our babies are having when we're on maternity leave with them, nor on any of the multitudinous and understandable anxieties that looking after a newborn brings. From the first round of jabs, to fevers spiking and random terrifying new things happening every day – like the first time I took our son to town and disembarked from the train wrongly and ended up getting the pram wheels stuck between the doors and the platform. (My heart leaped out of my body as my twelve-week-old baby dangled over the platform, people rushed to help and I felt deeply embarrassed as well as so very scared.) It's a mistake I have never repeated and a lesson I've never forgotten, to always reverse off the train when pushing a pram or buggy, stepping down first with the back wheels. But it still haunts me.

I am not going into this, even though it's a crucial part of the mental soundtrack playing on a loop during this period, because my aim is to try to distil as faithfully as I can the part of maternity leave that's about the mother's reaction to this unique time. Not her reaction to her child.

You may relate to my dispatches from the maternity front line. You may not. You might fall somewhere in the middle. All I am hoping for is that I might encourage you to enter this new and strange (and sometimes wonderful) land with your eyes wide open for its pitfalls as well as its peaks.

RENAME
AND
RECLAIM

The concept of maternity leave gathered steam during the Second World War as women went to work in a whole new way and nurseries were established to answer the urgent need for formalized childcare.

But, amazingly, maternity leave didn't become a mainstream political issue until well into the seventies and eighties as the law struggled to keep pace with social change. It's still a struggle to marry the two – despite fifty-two weeks' leave being technically permitted – because of the pay (or lack thereof), the paucity of decent and affordable childcare and barely veiled maternity discrimination.

In one important sense maternity leave is a misnomer, as it involves no actual leave. You are constantly on. Even when your offspring is having a nap, you are gearing up for their next appearance, or on alert for their first whimper before the big cry. Whether it's prepping bottles, doing the endless laundry, planning out the afternoon – where the feed might happen, where you might find nappy-changing facilities as well as somewhere for you to take a pee yourself – there is nothing restful about it.

In another sense, maternity leave is aptly named, although I suspect not in the way it was originally intended. It's a period of leave from all you know: taking leave of one's mind, body, job and relationships.

So I propose an urgent renaming for the sake of accuracy. We insist upon such things with other roles in life ('housewife' and 'spinster', I'm looking at you). At this moment in time, when you've just officially named the human you have created, you are arguably more aware than at any other point of the fact that names matter. And this is about much more than just wordplay. Renaming maternity leave might truly help better prepare women for what is to come.

I say that 'maternity leave' should be no more. Instead, we should call it 'maternity *service*'. Deep breath and repeat. Maternity service.

Think about it, especially if you've already experienced it for yourself: there are the same repeated duties, day in and day out; lots of kit that needs to be acquired and mastered (and often lugged around); full-body workouts; night shifts that turn into day shifts; an unofficial uniform; a plethora of injuries; the sense of unrelenting effort for a larger, not always fully comprehensible long-term goal and then the slow satisfaction that comes from doing your bit – for your baby and your family.

You are *serving* – your baby, your growing family, yourself – as you nurture your nearest and dearest. The definition of service is the act of helping someone. An alternative word for service is 'kindness'. Loving service is just that. And this is a huge part of this period in your life. But such a rebrand also makes room to reflect the sheer drudgery, tedium and downright shitty parts of it too.

Different people do different lengths of maternity service tours. If society likened looking after your newborn to more like a job of duty (albeit fuelled and imbued with the greatest love there is) – almost like one long Duke of Edinburgh's Award scheme, the Brownies or the military – it would be a better and more accurate way to describe what actually goes down.

'Duty' is not a fashionable word these days. But I am a fan. Certain things just have to be done in all of our lives, so learning to carry on carrying on, without rebelling or overthinking, is a valuable skill. Not one I've particularly mastered, I should hasten to add. But this type of deep acceptance and the realization that all you are doing during maternity service is a means to an end – you have a baby to have a child to have a family, that's the destination – is a helpful reality check when you find yourself deep in the newborn trenches. This being my second tour, the concept of duty definitely helped me do better at accepting the trudge rather than fighting it, which is what I wasted a lot of time and energy on the first time around.

There is also a useful stoicism that comes with the idea of service and duty. In a world filled with people talking about the search for purpose and meaning, often from the perspective of how to improve only one person's life, namely your own, 'duty' speaks to a bigger purpose. To community and how we all fit together. You haven't only grown a baby, you have grown a person, and maternity service will, amazingly, end up being only a very small part of this process.

All of this healthy perspective will disappear, of course, when you haven't slept and can't seem to leave the house without another fluid explosion from your baby's mouth or bum or both, but it is a framework upon which to re-angle the whole 'mat leave' idea. And one you can return to when times are tough.

And it helps to remember that, like all periods of service, it will come to an end.

The very idea of service, something usually associated with the military, might help you dig deep in very difficult moments, as well as encouraging you to lean on others, if you can, for the support you need. Just as a soldier would lean on their sisters-in-arms. By contrast, maternity 'leave' just sounds too gentle and like you're on some kind of relaxing break.

This time around I have properly leaned into this concept of service and duty as a core part of my survival, especially with ill health blighting my path, courtesy of endometriosis and the physical pain it can cut into you. And it has helped me to imagine this tour of duty I find myself on again as made up of some of the aspects of military service: duty, sacrifice, a uniform, war wounds, sisters-in-arms, discipline, battle fatigue and, above all, a sense of mission.

You could think of the pages that follow as being a little like a service manual. After all, having a baby is like setting off a bomb in your life – a love bomb, but one that still has a hell of an impact – so this is my attempt to carve a path through the chaos, however wayward. And to provide a hand of friendship that I would have truly appreciated. While I was lucky to have some wonderful sisters-in-arms – we were newbies together – I know it would have made a difference to have had someone sending dispatches from deep inside the fog of new motherhood. Before their experience was sanitized or misremembered.

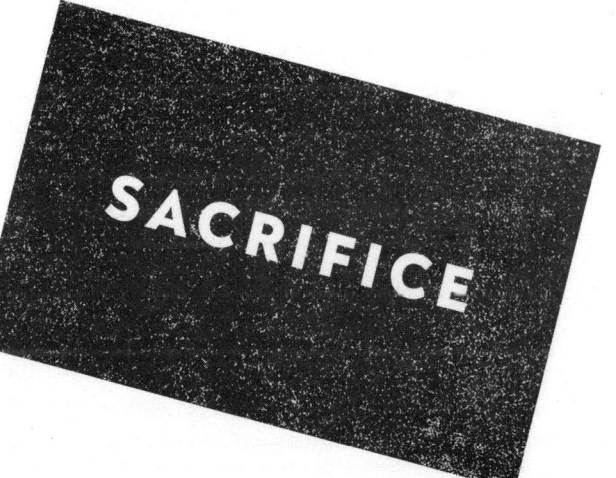

Maternity service is an exercise in extreme patience. I don't mean with the baby – that comes later, when they become toddlers. I mean for your needs and desires. You might think of something simple but necessary that you want to do for yourself, like buy a blister plaster, but it might take a week until you a) remember and b) manage to order it online or get to a shop. This paragraph has ironically taken three days to write since I first thought to mention one of the hallmarks of maternity service: deferred gratification – the parking of personal desires until later in the day or several weeks or months on. This in itself is a good skill to nurture. But, my god, it takes some adapting to.

Delayed gratification is so extreme during maternity service that although it's something that continues in one form or another as your baby gets older, those later stages will seem tame by comparison. Never mind not being able to poo alone or on your own schedule – one sometimes can't even poo *in* the loo. The author Natasha Lunn wrote of her recent mat service: 'One day I even shat myself, not out of martyrdom, but because I didn't have time to go before I left the house and then Joni [her eldest] decided to have a tantrum on the street and I couldn't carry her home because I was already carrying Vega [her newborn], so . . .'

Take today: as a keen litter picker, sadly rarely out of business in London, I have walked past the same heap of rubbish – a mix of clothes, chicken bones and food wrappers due to high winds – three times in the last twenty-four hours. But I have been unable to go and get my litter claw to scoop it up in a bag as I have either been on my way to walk the screaming baby to sleep or rushing home to retrieve her milk or put her down for a longer nap. Once I am home, I can't nip out with my trusty claw and do it then as I won't be able to leave the baby. Something so mundane, fast and satisfying is totally out of reach until my husband is home, and by then I might have completely run out of the mental and physical fuel required to go and do it as night falls. Or I might not. I might be fired by a small spark of independence. The point is that right now I just don't know which it will be. It's a small example, but ponder it for a moment, the cumulative effect of moments like this on one's brain and sense of self. It's a tiny act that would serve myself and the community around our street. And I can't do it. Despite knowing how much I want to.

So it slides. In my regular life, this wouldn't usually even merit much thought, let alone be considered worthy of being written down. Yet on maternity leave it becomes, like so much else, another thing that needs to be planned and is then all too often abandoned. Something dangled just out of reach. And it is this complete lack of agency that I want to bear witness to, because it's one of the reasons why some women's lights can diminish for a while on maternity leave or, worse, slowly go out.

The other day I had the radio on, Radio 4 in this instance

(a rarity on my maternity leave as it's just too weird to listen to your place of work, and I also end up shouting questions and thoughts at it), and a very successful male artist was talking about why he keeps on working. I kid you not, it went something like this: 'I work because I must have purpose and it would be my worst nightmare to wander about alone with my thoughts all day.'

I sat upright from where I had been playing with my baby on her playmat and laughed ruefully, replying aloud: 'Mate, you just described maternity leave!'

Also, know this, Mr Artist: YOU CAN HAVE A THOUGHT OR AN IDEA ON MATERNITY LEAVE AND YOU MIGHT NOT BE ABLE TO MAKE IT HAPPEN FOR TWO WHOLE WEEKS. Yes, you have to keep thoughts or ideas warm until, like my litter-picking, there is a snatched moment to execute them.

It shouldn't be underestimated how frustrating and deadening it is not to be able to achieve anything tangible in the day. Even the smallest of things.

Deadening. It's an odd word to use when you are in the process of looking after a life right at its very start. But the effect on the mother, who is often very tired indeed, can be a deadening one as the same tasks are performed daily while their own plans are put to one side. And their old life slips out of view. Albeit temporarily.

It is also important to remember that we women doing maternity service have already been delaying our own gratification during nine months of pregnancy, as our body became a vessel for another body and our baby's needs came to the fore. Every move we made or food we ate was considered through the lens of how it affected someone else. In my case this dance had been going on for two and a half years before my pregnancy even started, thanks to a cocktail of IVF drugs and living a life of near abstinence.

So thinking of this whole experience as maternity *service* really helps, because you can embrace the idea of self-sacrifice – while also remembering that this near erasure of self does not and will not be permanent.

And I appreciate there will be people reading this who say, go figure, you've had a kid. Count yourself lucky. This shunting of your own needs far down the pecking order is just how it is. I know that. And I also know it's a finite experience. But it is still, for many of us on maternity service, a new and unsettling experience, and my hope is that it might help others going through the same period if I can share how it feels at the time.

I wish I was better at smiling beatifically and being satisfied 24/7 with baby gurgles and snuffles and nuzzles. And it's true that in those first early months a big part of me wanted to nurse, heal and nurture, and be in my newborn bubble – with all the delayed gratification that came alongside it. But now that the first six months are done and breastfeeding is over for me, something I read recently about Angelina Jolie comes to my blurred mind. She said she was drawn to action movies when the early newborn days were done as she had been all soft and mumsy and she craved something hard and tough. She needed the contrast and to feel physically strong. I personally feel right now like I am held together with string. And at times even that is fraying as I am still recovering physically and emotionally. But I totally relate to needing that contrast and reclaiming of oneself.

I need grit and laughter. I want to go hard. Go party. Go travelling. Get strong and healthy and fit. Anything to rip the Band-Aid off, dial back the self-sacrificing and be me. But we are where we are and that is not to be. Yet.

In the meantime, you need to do whatever it takes to get through it, and take the wins where you can find them.

A lot of maternity service is about holding one's nerve – especially when it comes to matters of sleep (theirs *and* yours). Moreover, it's about learning to trust your own judgement, and this isn't easy when you are often operating in a climate of fear, especially when it's your first baby, against a backdrop of intermittent screaming and your own desperation for more shut-eye. Fear you are getting it wrong; fear the baby is not going to be all right; fear things will never improve; fear your life may not be recognizable again. All of this fear is imbued with a new love, which raises the stakes still higher. I often can't hear my own thoughts until the baby stops screaming and only then can I remember to breathe and think normally again. And this is my second child. It's umbilical.

Just as military recruits are trained to operate in hostile environments, you need to be ready to dig deep at times and carry out tasks against a backdrop of chaos. It may be domestic chaos but it's still a challenge to navigate.

It helps if you can learn to back yourself, even if all of the signs sometimes point in the other direction. Just recently I roared like an Olympian bagging gold when I found myself on one of the hottest days of the year walking our screaming daughter around a cobbled square in front of art students, having hastily evacuated the Tate Britain cafe. I did around ten laps and she went back off to sleep for a further ninety minutes. Yes, I was dripping with sweat. Yes, I'd abandoned my friend. But my instincts had been right. She just needed more sleep. I held my nerve and a great daytime nap ensued.

Whether it's making a judgement call about when your screaming baby must sleep despite all of the odds seeming stacked against you achieving that in the public space you find yourself in, or politely ignoring well-meaning 'advice' from strangers which can be just wrong as it might relate to different scenarios, learning to trust your own instincts also really helps restore your sense of who you are. Just because you're trying to embrace the idea of self-sacrifice, it doesn't mean you need to outsource your judgement to everyone around you or lose faith in your own decision-making skills – especially as you get to know your baby. And yourself, again. Some of you is still in there and having faith in your own decisions can be a vital reminder of that reality.

UNIFORM

Maternity leave can seem as though it is almost designed to make you not feel like *you* – on the outside just as much as the inside.

Reflecting on my first maternity tour, I realize I found it helpful to equip myself with a uniform, right down to keeping the same hair bobble, with just enough stretch, always on my wrist, ready to sweep away my long hair at a moment's notice for breastfeeding or bouncing the baby so he couldn't grab at it and more pain ensue. I even slept with it on – despite my loathing of wearing any jewellery in bed – because this is a job where you need to be ready to roll at all hours. I discovered that wearing a long open shirt over any jumper or T-shirt was flattering to my slowly deflating body with all its new lumps and bumps. Remarkably, the same fraying long denim shirt that survived my first tour has reappeared like an old friend for this one. I find I like the hole that's growing on the left elbow, threatening to rip open – just like its owner, emotionally and physically, post birth. Denim has both the hardiness and style I am looking for. Fingernail deep in baby shit and nappy rash cream, I am not messing about. This shirt, and two more replicas, basically act as a modern-day housecoat.

A uniform is also far more commensurate with the idea of maternity service, as opposed to the softer-sounding 'maternity leave'. And a hardy uniform at that, ready for all kinds of spillages and leaks.

I see other women adopting the same strategy during our daily trawls of the neighbourhood park or baby classes at the local church, council hall or gym. Long baggy T-shirts, hair scraped back and stretchy trousers – perhaps a jaunty scarf or two – as well as sweatshirts with ironic slogans bought by well-meaning pals to keep morale high: GOOD MUMS SAY BAD WORDS, or IF MY MOUTH DOESN'T SAY IT, MY FACE DEFINITELY WILL.

During the winter months of the first part of this maternity tour, I took the reins and, channelling my inner Steve Jobs, bought the same black stretchy polo neck four times over and wore the same two pairs of maternity jeans on rotation. I could breastfeed in my uniform and it was very, very flattering – which made me feel a bit better about myself. There were only three feeding bras too, so no thought was needed for the undergarments either.

Since then, during the summer months, I have worn the same style tunic dress that I bought three more of and I wear them on repeat. These are clothes that don't make me feel too shit. And ones I can breastfeed in too. And then there's the fact that I can actually fit into them – that was basically the bar.

A uniform is also something you are given to wear for a job, something suitable, often temporary and definitely not *you*. It helps you perform your role. And while this makes sense, it doesn't mean it isn't boring or frustrating. Thinking about how I dress has been a key part of how I have communicated my identity to myself and others since I was fourteen. Now I must dispense with these thoughts to avoid losing time I don't have, and I must engage with a body that isn't the one I am familiar with. In some ways you could argue it's freeing. But despite that truth, I still can't wait for the day when I put all my maternity uniform away or donate it to the next mother at the charity shop – if it's serviceable after several very hot washes.

The plus side to a uniform is that you can style and tweak it to your needs, because it's an aesthetic based mainly on how it helps you perform your role. What's often far, far harder is how to re-find yourself aesthetically away from the role. Later, I will return to the idea of not looking – and therefore not feeling – like yourself during this stage of your life and how you might need to prepare for that in other ways.

ROUTINE
(DRILL TIME)

For me, routine, preparation and planning wherever I can has been key to *getting on* getting on during maternity service.

Every night, since stopping breastfeeding, I try to wash and prep all the bottles for the next day – or my husband does. I put out my washed (if I remember) water bottle on the mantelpiece near the front door so I don't forget my own means of hydration.

I also empty the pram of as much debris as I can be bothered to in a bid to be set up for the morning. There are rain covers, waterproofs for me and an umbrella. When the sun started to come out, a picnic rug was added to the bottom carriage – which has become like a mini house for me. And if anyone messes with the household contents, it's not pretty.

Every weekday morning, come rain or sun, regardless of how little sleep has been had, I try my hardest to be out of the front door by nine a.m. at the latest. That's my drill time. Even if I have nowhere to go – though I usually try to have at least one job or person in the schedule to hang the day around – the minute my foot hits the pavement we are back in the world. On those days when I don't have anything planned to make me open the door, I feel the impact. Having a plan makes everything just a little bit more anchored and real. I feel better; more purposeful. Plus, I got out! I still want to scream with joy and high-five any mother I see out on the street with a very small baby and say, 'WELL DONE. YOU DID IT. YOU GOT OUT.'

The nine a.m. exit has become a sacrosanct ritual. A goal in a goalless space. As has my ten a.m. cup of tea. It's my mid-morning check-in, tethering me to the strings of the real world. Hitting these daily targets – however out of reach they have been at times – and sticking to my self-created routine has become a vital part of my maternity service.

And then there's the walking. Right now, I am averaging 12–14,000 steps a day. I am like an explorer with nothing to find. A slightly new route or the discovery of something I've never seen before in the miles surrounding my house can yield disproportionate excitement. A few weeks ago I discovered a WHOLE NEW CUL-DE-SAC I never knew existed. Yes, it contained a gift shop and a coffee place I had never heard of, but those lovely things paled in comparison to the find that was a female-owned independent wine-tasting bar, also serving the most delicious snacks and, wait for it, hosting maternity-leave tastings. The woman who owned this nirvana remembered the desert that was maternity leave and, having clawed her way out, vowed to never forget the land she'd left. Her Friday maternity tastings were born and I was in. All in.

After booking one the very next week, with one of my two sisters-in-arms on this tour of duty, we did mums the world over proud. School pick-up on foot and by bus that day was definitely bouncy. I was asleep/passed out by eight p.m. that evening.

Obviously there have been days, weeks even, when all of these 'get out of the house by nine' plans have fallen to shit. Utter shit. Sometimes, literally, because of a shit. One day we couldn't move for the stuff. But then humour is also essential for a life of service. And poo war stories really do provide some of the best material for the rest of your life. You will never forget the day you caught your kid's poo in a bread bag. Ever.

But you try your very best to start again. Over and over. You might not be able to hear the rhythm of the other millions of women doing exactly the same the world over in the first few days, weeks and months of a baby's life, but be comforted by the idea that you are marching in lockstep, sometimes joyfully, sometimes tearfully. Sometimes utterly vacantly.

And while making sure you try not to miss the window to get out is a key part of the drill, an equally important part is what you do with your time – and how you think about it – when you come back in.

If you manage to get the baby to nap in the house – in the buggy by the door or in their cot (the absolute jackpot) or anywhere else that works for you – perhaps a particularly small loo with good daytime blackout vibes? – then you can seize this golden opportunity to just *be*. Or you can run around getting jobs done if that helps you feel less consumed by chaos. Despite all the advice, I know few women who are able to actually 'nap when baby naps', outside of those first few weeks. And even then it feels rare – so please don't beat yourself up if napping is not something you can fit into your drill.

Another friend swears by doing nothing when their baby naps beyond reading a book. Ideally outside if it's good weather, or at least by a window.

The golden rule seems to be that whatever you choose to do in these precious moments, DO NOTHING you are able to do when the baby is awake. So, if you can stop yourself (and I know it's hard), don't try and deal with the endless laundry or do the washing-up or start prepping the next meal. When the baby sleeps, only do things you genuinely *can't* do when the baby is awake. Like reading a book. Or planning something you can look forward to on the computer or your phone – something you need a present, undistracted mind for. Or having a bath – but be ready to be pulled out of it quickly! Mindless tasks or chores, albeit often requiring two hands, should only be done when your baby is awake and with you, and you can split your attention. Putting away the never-ending piles of laundry is chief amongst them.

The same friend told me she was suspicious if a woman on maternity leave's home was suddenly spotless. That's not what is meant to be happening. I struggle a little with this because, for me, a tidy place does mean a tidier mind, and on my first maternity service, I found myself tidying mostly in an attempt to achieve *something*. This mat leave? I have decided to think of it almost like a feminist protest. Why should I do all of the household tasks simply because I am the one at home? I am helping the newest member of the family to be. *That* is the job. And it's the core of my drill.

WALKING
WOUNDED

Maternity service is nails. No other job requires you to go into it injured. Not even the military expect that. Match fit is usually a basic requirement.

But, by contrast, many women often begin their maternity tour expecting a soft, cocooning time filled with only gurgles, sniffs of that glorious new baby-head smell and dreamy kisses. There are those moments, of course – and they get you through – but there is a heck of a lot else that's hard, loud and messy all around the edges. And utterly, utterly knackering.

Lack of sleep should not be underestimated as a key and constant companion to the new you. We don't realize how powerful sleep is until we lose it. It is actually the stuff of magic, and it can transform the same experience from a nightmare into a dream – and vice versa. How a night has gone with your baby can make all the difference in the world.

Lucy Jones brilliantly describes these newborn nights as 'anarchic'. She writes: 'I am bruised by fatigue. I'm breastfeeding 18 times a day, for an hour each time. "That's wonderful," I'm told, as I slip into nervous exhaustion.' Cluster feeding? More like cluster fuck.

There is a reason sleep deprivation is used as a form of torture. And this is one particular ride you can't get off because it's now YOUR LIFE. Enduring broken night after broken night, and the bone-deep tiredness that comes from them, alters you in ways you cannot comprehend and diminishes your capacity for straight thought and proportionate reactions to things that normally might not even make you blink. Sleep deprivation makes people thin-skinned and can lead to severe mood-plummeting moments. A new friend told me, upon thinking back to her first tour, how stunned she had been by the change that only a few days of little sleep wrought in her. Now, layer a few more weeks and then months on top of that and you can understand why she compared her sleepless scratchy self to a snail without a shell.

Lack of sleep also significantly reduces one's abilities to understand the basics and to see the bigger picture. As soon as someone gives me a clear run at my bed, I am born anew. Even a twenty-minute power nap can reverse a dark day so that it feels suddenly lighter. Ironically, although I have never before been more aware of each of the many minutes that make up a day, I have also learned that the more hours I spend awake in the world, the less I understand it.

And then there are the post-natal complications.

In my case, my herniated disc actually came on eight weeks post-partum as I have zero core strength after two C-sections. But it was during a bad bend to get the baby out of her bouncer, the morning after I went for a gentle swim to start to help myself, that my back just went and I hit the deck, aka the cool tiled floor next to our loo. I learned too late that keeping my head out of the water, due to my poor eyesight, as I did breaststroke for twenty lengths had been possibly the worst way to position my spine.

I am now resigned to physiotherapy and a life of Pilates. And slow recovery. Very slow. It's so upsetting. I've sobbed, I've raged, and I am learning again to be patient. It's not my husband's fault, but this hasn't happened to him. And he doesn't have a myriad of physical issues to fix and heal from – which can at times feel like they need an entire maternity leave of their own – from a hypertonic pelvic floor to wondering whether you can ever sneeze safely again.

And then there are the moments that raise your game to a whole other level. Breastfeeding through the pain of mastitis or a slipped disc is other-worldly horrible. Or a scary doctor's appointment or a trip to A&E for the baby, when suddenly nothing in the whole world is right and you find yourself making deals with any god who might be willing to listen that you will give anything, anything, for your baby to be safe and well.

In all these times when there isn't any other way but through, thinking of maternity leave as my own personal tour of duty has helped me grit my teeth and breathe, knowing that millions of other women are also digging deep and trying to safely navigate around their own tender bodies as well as the new tiny body they are responsible for. I try and remember how the endless backdrop of sleeplessness can also make you laugh crazily and love hot drinks more than is humanly possible. And how it forms a bond with your fellow mat-leave sisters in a way that you won't recognize once you leave this land.

I imagine all the other walking wounded mothers battling on, collecting hard-earned scars, and find myself in awe of this strength that comes from having something so defenceless in your charge.

SISTERS-IN-ARMS

I liken maternity service to one big radio show for which I have to cast the guest list, hour by hour. Yes, I know radio is my normal job, but it's a personal work comparison which might help you too as you find yourself walking the streets aimlessly and in need of adult company. Let me explain.

I begin my roll-call by making a list of all the people I know who might be available to meet up, and I work my way through it. And then I start getting increasingly random and looking up all sorts of people who might, possibly, like to see me and the baby, and who might be free. I would go so far as to say I am a social slut on maternity leave. I even asked for the phone number of one startled woman I had met only once at a mother-and-baby class because she smiled at me and I realized I was running out of walking partners. I followed up with a text but she has yet to reply . . . what can I say? I am a geriatric millennial (born in 1985), while she seemed younger and probably found me overly forward on the communication front.

But the irony is – and this is the one I still struggle to get used to – that most of the social time you spend with other adults while you're on maternity leave can be quite rubbish. It is an exercise in lowering expectations. Recently I had a cousin visiting from abroad. We met for breakfast at a lovely place I'd booked. Old me would have been excited to hear about her life. New me wanted her to see the baby, see me, eat some food and then for us all to get out in one piece. I spent the whole time we were together firstly bouncing the baby post-feed as she cried, then trying to clean up after she was sick on me and on my cousin, and generally getting myself very sweaty. I heard about three things my cousin said. We got the photo, said our goodbyes and out of there I flew to get home in time for the afternoon nap.

It almost wasn't worth it. Almost. But what else was I going to do? It passed some time and broke the monotony of the day; I wanted my daughter to meet my wider family, I wanted to see my cousin, and, despite all the baby sick and sweatiness and our inability to finish any sentences, it was still a memorable experience.

But oh, the relief once I was out of the restaurant and my daughter could just cry it out alone! Immeasurable. Plus, I didn't need to expend any more of my flagging energy trying to listen, talk, eat and placate. I loathe not being able to be the best version of myself – telling funny stories and receiving them in kind. Even remembering to compliment friends and family is just not happening right now. But again I have learned to try and accept this. Grudgingly.

Maternity service is a time that is filled with moments like this, when you think that for the effort expended to get somewhere – and then how challenging it ended up being – you almost shouldn't have bothered. But most of the time you were right to try, and the experience of nearly not doing it and *then* doing it? That's what adds texture and shine to it all. *That* is the line you live on.

And therein lies a central rub of maternity leave: you often can't be with people but you can't be without them either. The whole social side of it is a bizarre, frustrating, bonding and utterly maddening exercise in unfinished thoughts, laughing, sharing war stories and walking, so much walking . . .

The best people to recruit alongside you on this march are those who are in the exact same situation as you are, so nobody minds when you suddenly have to leave or break off in the middle of a sentence. Or those who don't have children with them when you meet and so can be another pair of hands – if they are willing.

You don't need a full squad of new mothers, although it's lovely if you find one. Just one sister-in-arms will be enough. I have had a few key women get me through each of my maternity services; one I still refer to as my mat-leave wifey. She became a second spouse as we got through the days together. Another of my squad mates I called 'Soldier', as she did me. We still only address each other as such to this day.

In the exercise class I mentioned at the start of this book, where I felt the fire in my belly to break ranks, I was one of only two second-time mothers in the room. Interestingly, we were both the most honest in our introductions to the group, as she quietly talked of her prolapse and lowered her aching body down on to the mat with a small wince, all the while soothing her baby. I was grateful for her frankness, which helped cut through the feeling that we were all playing a role in some weird war movie in which we'd been told to keep buggering on and not to mention the battle that had just physically and emotionally ravaged us.

Once I'd said my piece, another woman (who was absolutely living the dream – attending a mother-and-baby exercise class without her baby as her husband was on the latest doctors' strike and was caring for their little one at home, so she could actually do some post-natal fitness) eventually piped up: 'I find alcohol really helps! It's the only way to get through.'

And we all laughed. Because we knew what she meant. A little drink or three in the day with friends massively helped me last time. And it has done again. But if alcohol isn't your tipple, then tea or cake or coffee – or whatever takes your fancy to share in together – helps with laughing more, passing the time more joyfully and forging new bonds with women who suddenly come into your life, if you are lucky, simply because you procreated at the same time. Or, in my case, injected IVF drugs at a similar time. It's the same randomness with which we make some of our most important friends at school and university – we just happen to be the same age because our parents bonked in the same twelve-month window.

Recently, I watched with joy two very unlikely women meet for a mother-and-baby class and collapse into listening to each other's experiences, gratefully exchanging the smallest details about their babies' respective nights and their own. I found it very moving to observe the intensity of this shared bond; a life raft in a sea of uncertainty, between two women who you could tell would never have found each other in their normal lives, and who now cleaved to one another in a way only women do. I cannot imagine men, as much as they need their friends, talking their experience out in this way, minute by minute, whether in person or online during the night shifts.

While much has rightly been written and said about the isolation of new mothers – as we raise our children more and more alone, holed up in flats and homes away from the old support networks – we shouldn't overlook the new networks women manage to form to get them through this time.

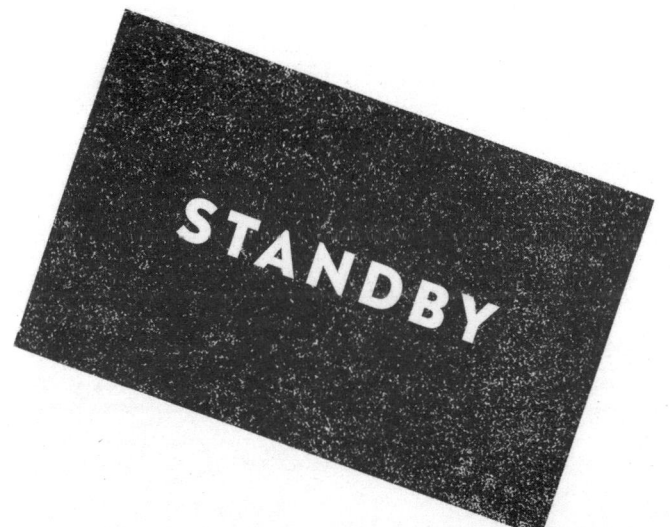

The time has come for me to try and describe the ineffable: the all-encompassing boredom of maternity service. But boredom is too passive a word to describe a situation in which you are busy but your mind is not. You aren't at a loss for what to do – but the things you are doing are largely the same hour by hour, and life doesn't quicken or alter in quite the jagged way it does in your 'regular' existence.

There have been days when I have waited for the moment I needed to leave for the school pick-up for our five-year-old – after I have fed the baby and prepped an after-school snack and the evening's bottles and dinner – and I have genuinely spent that time watching the hands of the kitchen clock, as there wasn't enough of a window in which to go for a walk or fit anything else in. I don't think I have ever known the inside of a minute quite so intimately before. I felt every one of those sixty seconds of every minute that passed.

And yes, I know the actual job of keeping a baby alive and thriving – as well as teaching them to safely roll, sit, touch and taste – is HUGE. The biggest. And the most important – even if society has made us feel it is anything but. But it's happening so, so, *so* slowly, you don't get that buzz or change of pace most humans crave from their day. The contrasts are so small they are barely perceptible. And yet compare this to the experience of a grandmother who pops in every now and then, or even a partner who comes back to the baby after a day at work. The contrasts seem so much larger for them as they get to leave, live their lives and return. And the act of leaving, for many, many hours, gives them an energy and perspective the one left behind simply cannot share. Understandably, this makes them coo with excitement if even the smallest development has happened. They have so many other things going on in their lives that suddenly being with the baby, like sweets given in moderation, becomes an exciting treat.

The business of maternity service also doesn't fill your entire mind. Your brain is being used very differently – and it's a whole-body job – leaving you knackered at the end of the day, on top of the mind-altering sleep deprivation. But there are many minutes in that day when you long for something else to occupy your consciousness, something, anything, more nourishing than your own thought loop and the constant task list. Even narrowly missing being clipped by a bicyclist who ran a red light the other day gave me an adrenaline buzz I'd missed. As I shouted after him out of shock and fear I felt a surge of electricity run through my body and I almost relished it.

I liken existing on maternity leave to being an appliance on standby mode. I am here but not fully. And sometimes I flick on and experience a gorgeous high I will remember forever – like the first giggle of our son at six months, which erupted from nowhere. I still regularly relive it, mentally savouring the moment, thrilled I didn't miss it. But there were many, many minutes in that day alone, never mind the preceding six months, in which NOTHING happened and I just had to be alone with my thoughts, doing domestic drudgery and Groundhog Day tasks.

Or the other day when our daughter cut her first two teeth without any fuss at all and I suddenly spied these two gleaming white stumps on her bottom gum through her smiling lips. I squealed and wished her congratulations. Her smile grew even wider, the apples in her delicious cheeks bigger, as she buzzed off my excitement. That buzz continued for me for at least four hours. But before that, I had been chopping veg, tidying, changing nappies, feeding and prepping for the school run and double bedtime routine for THREE HOURS and nothing had happened.

This is why I want to send a message to any older woman who feels compelled to say something like this to new mothers: 'Make the most of every second. Enjoy every minute, it goes so fast. I wish I could have my time again with my little ones' – *Please don't*. Even though you mean well, it's the most maddening and unhelpful piece of advice.

I am living every second. Truly. In a way I have never experienced time before. Time is practically bending before me. That bloke on Radio 4 spoke truth about not being able to hack this amount of time alone with one's thoughts. And I promise you I am here for every second. Every single one. But it is impossible to enjoy every second of anything. Never mind in this strange liminal land that is maternity leave. Telling us to do so places a whole other pressure on us that we don't need.

I have developed a theory that it's almost impossible to fully savour the experience of your babies at the time they are babies because you will always miss them being babies. You just will. It's hard-wired into us. All you need to know is you were there. They were there. And somehow you muddled through. And it's fine not to enjoy all of it. Or even much of it. But know that you grabbed the bits that you did and try very hard to remember how it felt to hold the whole of your child in your arms and those fleeting gorgeous moments when they put their head into the nape of your neck.

As for the woman who I referred to in my introduction, who recently looked baffled when I said I find maternity leave largely dull and boring, and who unintentionally made me feel awful when she replied: 'Oh really? I was never bored – you have so much to do looking after the children' . . . I just smiled through gritted teeth. She couldn't understand what I was trying to express. Nor would she have listened if I'd wearily tried to defend myself against her judgement of me. Of course I am busy with exactly the same parenting jobs she had. But it doesn't mean my mind is busy. And that's what dictates my boredom levels. Not what my hands can now almost do with my eyes closed. So instead of explaining this, I just smiled at her and looked down at my baby girl (who I am convinced shared my point of view – she's my daughter, after all).

But a few days later, when I gently took on one of these well-meaning older mothers who became the fourth woman to tell me to enjoy every second, turning the tables and asking her to properly recall whether she indeed loved every part of her maternity leave, she paused, smiled sheepishly and said: 'No, no I didn't. I really didn't know what to do with myself other than find people to be with and go on endless, aimless walks. It was pretty odd and sad at times. But it wasn't about my daughter. It was me.'

Exactly, I thought. You. This is what this little book is trying to communicate. Something colossal that gets lost. How the woman navigates maternity leave. Not parenthood – although the two are linked – but rather this bewildering time out of regular life and into service.

After she said what she said, we both felt a bit better over a cup of tea in my local cafe – which we then switched to wine.

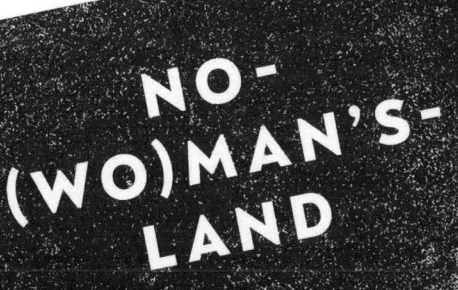

NO-
(WO)MAN'S-
LAND

One of the huge ironies of maternity service is that you are rarely alone. You are joined by the beautiful bean you've been waiting for. But because they can't give much back for a long time, it can feel very lonely. And this can happen as much when you are with other people as when you're by yourself.

Another conversation I happened to witness the other day at a mum-and-baby gathering perfectly summed up the difference between maternity leave and parenthood in general, and how crucial it is to delineate this experience – even with new friends.

One woman asked the other how she was getting on. It was clear they had only recently met through their babies. The other's entire answer was about her eleven-week-old baby, the sleep, her feeding and how many nappies she was getting through. The questioner's eyes glazed over. But she kindly forced herself to reply, offering comparable information about her baby's daily routine and habits in a bid to share and learn.

And that was that. It was as far as they went. Mainly because the responder was gushing and cooing about loving her baby so, so much – it drowned out any space for alternative experiences, even though it was so obvious the other woman was craving a totally different level of connection. This woman wanted to talk about herself, which became very obvious very quickly when I asked how she was doing at the end of the class and told her I was on my second maternity leave. Her reply?

One long exhale of air. Followed by: 'I am doing.' And then she almost whispered to me and my friend – feeling like weird veterans at this point, gearing up for the school run – 'It just doesn't feel like my life yet. And it's weirdly very long and dull, despite my loving my son so much.'

She then had to run back to her baby, before adding: 'I just didn't know it would feel like this.'

We did what we could to reassure her and there was a knowingness in our faces that seemed to calm her a little once she had escaped her pal.

Just knowing it's not only you is important.

SURVIVAL STRATEGIES

For those times when you find yourself desperately bouncing your baby, when food, nappy and sleep have all been tended to and yet they are still screaming – whether that's in the witching hour in the run-up to bedtime (if they even have one at this point) or at another moment during the day – I have found the following things can help take me out of myself.

A maternity service music playlist – to which you keep adding songs that you hear during this time – will help to just get you through. Dancing around with the baby, listening to tunes for *you*, somehow helps. Drowning out the crying is useful but also it allows you to distance yourself from the situation and stay calm. And it can make you smile too. Plus, it might even cheer the baby up. Such a playlist will also serve as a time capsule in the future that immediately carries you back to this mad and wonderful time.

But, crucially, music also allows you to access a part of yourself that is still unchanged from the land before – that you will get back to at some point – and restores a sense of self.

On mine right now I have: 'How This Came to Be' by Tom Rosenthal, 'Grounds for Divorce' by Elbow (I've reassured my husband that it's just a banging tune I need since hearing it anew on Apple's *The Morning Show*) and

Louis Armstrong's 'La Vie En Rose'. Like a magpie I have collected more than fifty songs during my service from podcasts I've trudged through rain to, box sets I've inhaled during afternoon feeds and cafe playlists I've drunk tea and bounced along to.

But for the moments when the screaming isn't stopping and perhaps you are out and about, and music cannot be played over a speaker, keep breathing and, if you can, develop a narrative over it. Talk loudly to your baby and make jokes. These are to cheer you up, calm you down and make others around laugh too – and show their solidarity – even if you feel mortified. Most people have been there and, even if they haven't, we were all babies once.

On my first maternity service, my new NCT pal Caroline was the best at this, cooing to her screaming son things like: 'I know! Mummy also needs a poo. I was just thinking that! What a great idea. Yes, I am also sad that so-and-so didn't win *Britain's Got Talent*' (or whatever the latest thing was she was watching). These quips allowed others in and made her feel less alone. It's way too easy to stop talking aloud to your baby – especially when you are on your own.

Wine. Beer. Gin. Whatever your poison. A word on it. I am not prescribing getting shit-faced every day, nor parenting completely addled. All in moderation. And again I know some people have real issues with alcohol themselves, or their parents did, which will inform their take on what I am about to share. But for me – a drink helps on maternity service. After the endless tea, a cheeky glass or two of wine in the afternoon with friends in the newborn trenches, or a mate who is willing to be there with you, is bliss.

Other forms of escapism are available and I should also mention the times when I have stayed indoors because of the herniated disc in my back or terrible weather or because I just couldn't be arsed to make a plan, and I have gone hard and deep into box sets. I binged so hard on Jennifer Aniston and Reese Witherspoon's *The Morning Show* I thought I worked on the set. The storylines permeated my mind asleep and awake. Equally, I strongly felt I was in line to succeed Logan Roy despite not being one of his moronic kids in *Succession*. And don't get me started on *The Marvelous Mrs. Maisel* and how I thought I too could make it as a Jewish comic in 1960s America . . .

I have also been to an early evening local dance session – booze free – and let myself go in that physical sense just to take the edge off. I escaped: my maternity duty, my mind and even my body. For two blissful hours. Urgently needed.

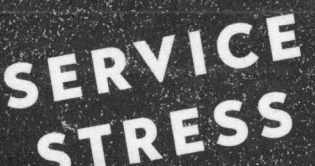

SERVICE
STRESS

I believe that at this moment in time Western women are the least prepared we have ever been for maternity leave and becoming mothers. We are being raised to shoot for the moon career-wise and share things equally with our partners if we have them. Then *wham bam* – maternity leave arrives. And, yes, it's an honour to be with your baby and see them slowly becoming their own person over the days and weeks, second by second. But it's also the first time many women find themselves putting their jobs in the deep freeze, carrying on with a joint project totally alone and doing the endless bloody laundry – even if partners do get a bit longer than two weeks or opt for taking shared leave. It's totally normal to be like: What. The. Hell. Is. This.

Enter rage. Simmering or full blast. Sometimes the rage is within, as you find yourself alone, again, at a social occasion, wheeling your baby as they fight against sleep, over some cobbles or down a side road away from sirens and other loud disturbances, while you DJ white noise on your phone, trying to balance it in the pram.

Or you have gone to a friend's house and, again, the baby needs to sleep and you can't quite make it work, screaming ensues, you can't concentrate on anything your pal is saying and you think you shouldn't have bothered – but equally you knew you needed to get out and be with people.

Or how about the time you have to make a swift exit from a gallery or museum because your baby is shrieking, cannot settle, and you suddenly have to leave your friend (whose baby will of course be sleeping peacefully) to find the nearest bit of rough road to try and bounce your own bub off to sleep.

None of your pals mind a jot by the way – but you do. And you aren't angry with the baby but with the situation and how, despite decent military-style planning, it's all gone to pot. You've ended up alone and with a very unsatisfactory social experience.

This rage may stay inside you, swirling around, like a persistent virus you can't quite vanquish, until one day it starts to dissipate. But it can also burst out. I have friends who have screamed into a pillow or just out loud – alone or in company – no longer giving a shit about who can hear them. Your co-colleague on maternity service screams with abandon – why not you? It makes total sense that a wildness might need to be unleashed.

Your partner, if you have one, has the same baby as you, and yet they look and feel almost exactly as they used to before its arrival. In my case, my husband is actually the fittest he's been for years. Meanwhile, I am the most destroyed I have ever been. Six months on, I feel like a truck has driven through me and my body.

It took me a while to locate the feelings of anger on my first tour, as I was just so shocked. Waving my husband off to work two weeks after I gave birth, barely standing, post C-section and breastfeeding around the clock, it was the first time in our relationship – and we have been together since uni – that something was genuinely not equal. The rage at the unequal distribution of labour arrived slowly but steadily, like a decent covering of snow – touching everything. I am usually a pragmatist and I believe in talking most things out until they are better, but I felt like I was being slowly mugged by a reality that had been there all along, unseen until now. And I was powerless to change it.

I also remember one day during that first tour when I silently handed our screaming son over to my husband as he walked in from work. I hadn't been able to soothe the baby for hours. I was wordless with fury at the world and marched off to KFC. I took it out on some hot wings and a mini fillet. I walked home, after a swift beer in the pub, and I don't think I spoke until two hours later. My husband looked at me with a quizzical yet nervous smile, wondering where his verbose wife had gone, but the eruption never came. The rage buried itself somewhere within – only to roar out of me some weeks later during my last bout of mastitis as I tried to dangle feed our child like a cow to get a dreaded lump out before a party. I was fully done.

Rage (and sometimes sorrow) are bound up in our relationships and our health, but also in how we look or don't look. Last week I ventured out on a shopping trip where I foolishly thought I'd try and buy a new dress to freshen up my wardrobe. I'd had the loveliest morning, buying some new shades and a fun cocktail ring just to brighten up my hands – the one part of me that hasn't changed too much (although I am still waiting for my wedding ring to fit again, so that's not entirely true). It was the first time I had bought anything new for myself in more than a year as I didn't want to acquire any more maternity clothes and had so far managed to stick to that resolution. And then I had to go and ruin it. The dresses either didn't do up or they didn't look how I'd imagined they would; I had chosen them for my old body and they looked all wrong on my new one.

My children had made me foreign to myself. I look down and don't recognize my body.

And yes, I know it takes time – but I genuinely didn't recognize the woman who came out of the changing room. It is incredible how different I looked in my mind to how I now look in reality.

Normally I pride myself on having a decent sense of humour and perspective – but this just felt shitty. I felt the same way once I'd finished breastfeeding, when I realized my old bras no longer fitted. 'Enjoy every minute!' they say. Does that include these minutes? At a time in your life when you are already struggling to feel like you, you also have to contend with the fact you no longer even *look* like the 'you' you were before.

A woman I know who never left maternity leave, staying at home to be with her two children full-time, recently went back to work after the best part of a decade away from her career. She stands by her choice for her and her family, but she talks powerfully of the fracturing she's survived: 'It's a literal metamorphosis for the woman. She is producing new people. There is the physical cracking of one's body and that's savage. But then comes the breaking apart of oneself emotionally. And then the rebuild job. It is as big as it gets,' she confides. She looks like she's seen some sides of life she'd really rather she hadn't.

It is all deeply discombobulating and frustrating, and the effects of this should not be underestimated. It also explains why so many women can't feel sexy, or don't like sex at this time in their lives. There is a new you. She might be staying. She might not. And she's so, so tired. And, sometimes, so, so angry about it all.

YOUR
MISSION

Maternity service is a time when you may find yourself hit by some massive existential questions: What is my life? How do I not just repeat my parents' lives – even if their lives are/were good? How can I be a good parent? And what do I want our lives to be now?

You are also dealing with now no longer being the youngest, the next generation. And this means you're suddenly looking at your life and what's happened up to this point, whether by design or accident, with new eyes. You're reassessing how things landed when the music stopped. On maternity service you are up very close to the cycle of life, with the result that you may find yourself wondering what it's all about and asking the big questions about how you want to use your remaining years.

Suddenly your job might not seem as important as it once did. Doubts about your set of beliefs – political, social, religious or otherwise – might emerge and demand your attention. You may find yourself overwhelmed by the facts of where you have ended up living, based on choices made long before you had considered how your existence might be with a little one in tow. It can all suddenly feel like *a lot*. This is the big heavy stuff that can come knocking during maternity service. But it is also perfectly understandable, as the tectonic plates keep slowly shifting beneath the land-scape of your world.

Try to talk it out and also perhaps just sit with some of those questions – or, more likely, walk with them. Pram-thinking once your baby is settled for a wee while is good time. Take these ports in the storm to ponder what you had perhaps been accepting without question before now. And see where it takes you. Or where it doesn't. And that's okay too. More than okay.

In one of my favourite *Woman's Hour* interviews, when I spoke with the amazing author Chimamanda Ngozi Adichie, we tried to articulate what motherhood does to the brain which leads to some of these new avenues of thought, and cuts off previously well-trodden neural path-ways. Chimamanda said that she has never gone back to who she was before having a baby. She also acknowledged that becoming a mother, even with all of the help she has, has deeply impacted her ability to write novels.

She knows. If you're reading this, perhaps you know? And in the interview, we did the best we could to commu-nicate from this far-off land, popping our heads above the trench to try to explain the unexplainable. Some might interpret this as complaining, but it isn't – it is articulating something which is important enough that it should have a dedicated correspondent on the nightly news. And yet it has never really been covered – because who has the words, time or inclination? This is why I am determined to try and find them.

In these many wobbly moments, those times when you find yourself adrift on an existential ocean, what I would say is: remember, your baby is your North Star. This might sound very, very obvious. But it's worth restating. Especially because when your face is pressed up against your stark new reality there's very little space to reflect on this.

While you are spending your every waking moment tending to their needs, it helps to recall that they are the reason you are in this swamp – wearing ill-fitting bras and stained clothes you vow to later burn. They are your mission. Use this thought as energy to get you through those testing moments as you try to find the pieces of yourself amongst the love rubble caused by the explosion of their arrival, and cling to it like your life depends on it. Because theirs does and therefore so does yours. Their thriving is the ultimate goal of this particular tour of duty. And, ironically, they will remember not a moment of it.

But *you* must remember this: there will still be time for you to make choices and changes and to find answers to the big questions that have bubbled up through the rubble. Nothing is set in stone. Don't lose sight of the fact that there is a long time *after* maternity leave – in the months and years that follow. You don't have to have the answers to these big, existential questions just now.

Breathe and repeat.

WHEN WILL MATERNITY LEAVE START?

I remember when our daughter was three months old and I met up with one of my friends in Birmingham. It was a big deal to get the train there from London and to find the right place to get on and off with the buggy. To add an extra frisson of danger to the proceedings, my daughter hadn't pooed for a week and the train changing table looked horrific. I was on edge but determined.

She is a wise and wonderful pal from school so I was resolute this was happening. I also wanted to see her nine-month-old and for our babies to meet each other. As it turned out – and rather hilariously – we didn't even leave Birmingham New Street train station as the changing facilities were amazing (even though no poo happened) and we essentially went on a restaurant crawl: three in one day between our trains.

But my mind keeps turning over something she said on that day, as she was coming to the end of her maternity service and I was just ramping up mine: she said she kept thinking during those nine months, *when* would her maternity leave actually start?

There was always something happening that made her feel like her leave hadn't quite begun. Major sleep issues, a minor medical issue, some setback with her health or with her baby's health, and on it went, never quite kicking off. And I know what she means. On maternity service, every time you crack something, something else cracks.

I keep thinking about this idea but then I try and remind myself that this is a strange and liminal time. Maybe, by definition, you will never quite feel that you've really got a handle on it. It's a bloody weird experience, maternity leave, and it's okay to acknowledge that. Remove anyone's daily routine, sleep, clothes, body, attention span, ability to complete thoughts and tasks, and it should be no surprise that they become completely discombobulated. And even when you do, finally, start to get more sleep, it is totally reasonable to find yourself thinking: what just happened?

One friend I spoke to recalled that on her maternity leave she had found the sensory and music classes for newborns rather perverse. Here was a group of slightly winded women trying to put a smile on their faces and keep themselves together singing nursery rhymes to babies who didn't really notice. She had been having a hard time at this point and found the whole thing darkly comic, as they all tried to make the best of suddenly finding themselves, as grown women, singing 'Twinkle, Twinkle, Little Star', sitting on the floor. She said it was like a scene out of a Stanley Kubrick film: bizarre, entertaining and slightly sinister all at the same time.

Personally, on my first maternity service, I found joy and structure in those classes but I also remember noticing how surreal the whole thing was; like it was we, the women, who had returned to childhood, singing songs to our babies instead of our dolls, trying to keep the whole show on the road. Who were the songs really for? The mothers or the babies?

Another mind-boggling aspect of maternity service is how unhealthy you can find yourself being, as you nail cake or deep-fried chicken at KFC (or in my case both), in full-on survival mode, while simultaneously wondering whether to purée carrot or sweet potato for your child's first taste of proper food. As you focus on the nutrients they need for healthy development, you've resorted to the anything-that-keeps-you-alive-and-sugared diet for yourself. (And if you are breastfeeding on this diet, there is another layer of irony in the mix too.)

And then of course, on top of all this, you feel guilty for not necessarily savouring the whole experience or loving every one of these minutes with your baby. Many of us simply can't – and I hope everything I've written within these pages will reassure you that this is okay too.

In the end, I think the only way to get your head around all of it is to remember that one of the reasons maternity service is so weird is because it was only ever designed to be temporary.

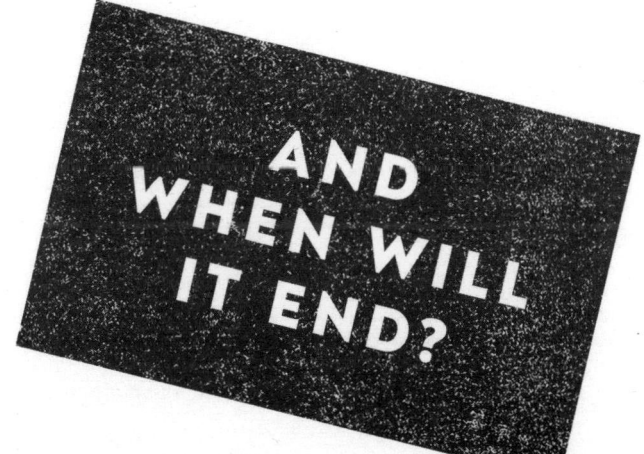

AND
WHEN WILL
IT END?

This is also the impossible question to answer. You go into maternity leave with one plan and then another one suggests itself almost immediately. On some days it can change minute by minute.

We need to make it easier to talk honestly about what the process of parenting – and specifically this initial and very intense probation period – actually feels like. It also needs to be possible to acknowledge the fact that not everyone is going to love it, at least not all of the time. It is totally natural to find much of it mind-numbing and a huge departure from what we might consider 'normal service'. Yes, there is your amazing baby right in the epicentre of this earthquake, but it is still an earthquake and an experience that would destabilize most people. Just as there are no long-service medals for extended maternity leave, those who opt for a shorter tour of duty should be able to feel that they can do so on their own terms.

If these conversations were more commonplace, perhaps we would feel more confident making the best decision about what kind of maternity leave to take and for how long. And more women might feel less ill-prepared and ill-informed.

While most women cannot easily afford to take a full year away from work, or even anything close to it, many do end up taking it, because they fear not getting this time again. Others feel that maternity leave starts to get more interesting once their baby is in the second half or last third of their first twelve months. Others may be unable to return to work because they are stuck in a loop of unaffordable – and all too often unavailable – childcare, or they may feel uncomfortable about their baby going into childcare too young. And for some, the knowing that twelve months is their right is another pressure in itself. They feel they ought to take it because it's allowed, and not doing so would somehow mean they weren't as dedicated to their child as they should be, and their baby would miss out.

So all I want to say on this point – while being mindful of how different people's situations and headspace can be about this – is that it's okay not to take twelve months' maternity leave. Truly. The only person judging and watching you is you. Interestingly, many of my older female friends, including one who is American and so comes from a country where the right to enough time away from work post-natally is far from ideal, often bemoan how extended maternity leave is in the UK. 'It's too long,' they declare, feeling that twelve months is too big a gap to take from one's job and one's identity. Their view is that women in this country can feel pressured to spend a year minimum with their child when actually a shorter time might suit them – in terms of what they need to feel like themselves again – and it wouldn't be to the detriment of the child. But too many women don't even entertain this idea because they have been made to feel like it is deeply wrong and transgressive.

The Irish writer Anne Enright once brilliantly wrote: 'Boredom is a productive state so long as you don't let it go sour on you. Try not to confuse the urge to get something done with the idea that you are useless.'

She wasn't talking about maternity leave but it works in this context too. Trying not to let maternity service go sour on you is a great goal. For my first tour I was out of the workplace for nearly eight months; my second will be nine months. Keeping sourness at bay is a challenge during the long days and nights. It is a finite time – and much of it is a precious time – but you still have to get through it. Minute by minute. Bottle by bottle.

Please try not to feel bad whatever you decide either way. I just hope you can feel that you had some sort of choice and the choice was driven by you.

THE
GREAT
RETURN

This period comes to an end. It really does. However long it ends up being for you, the tour of duty will come to a close. And you will return. You'll never be quite the same again. But you do return: reborn, blinking into the sunlight, wondering where the hell you've been.

I am writing this on the eve of my own 'returning'. Tomorrow I go back. Back to work. Back to before. Back to what?

I know I have a weird (but amazing) job that means I can't slink in behind a desk for the first few hours of being back at work after nine months 'off' and fly below the radar. Instead, my role means I open my mouth to a few million people and *go*. Whatever that will mean. Live broadcasting is one of my great loves because anything can, and does, happen. There's an alchemy unique to each day.

But like millions of other women when they return to work, it will still be highly performative.

In the last week, as I've approached this moment, I can feel it. The rose-tinted hue, the welcoming amnesia descending like a blanket over my maternity service. Muffling any cries of anguish and evening out the rough surfaces as reality passes into perfect fiction.

The French-Moroccan author Leïla Slimani said of motherhood that it is probably the 'most complex experience a human being can have but at the same time it's very disappointing . . . That sometimes makes me sad because I feel that everything people told me – especially my mother and grandmother – was partly a lie. We transmit lies to the next generation and maybe that should stop.'

I agree. These benign lies passed on from generation to generation in the Western world aren't a deliberate deception. In part they are because women don't want to hear the details of parenting until they are actually doing it. Which is fair enough. And when they do ask us, the women who have gone before them, for an honest account of maternity leave and beyond – we struggle to explain it. We partly gloss over the truth out of loyalty to and fierce love of our own beautiful babies. That's certainly my read on my own mother's totally rosy view of my perfect first year on earth – despite my arrival inducing some pretty awful post-birth injuries.

But mostly a fiction develops because it's so hard to remember, let alone articulate accurately, the experience of going on this strange journey into this strange land. With all this conscious and unconscious editing going on, the final script ends up pretty different to the first, very real draft.

How do you faithfully remember each of those minutes when the new keeper of your heart, your beloved baby, keeps distracting you with what feels like the final cuddles; the final morning walk; the final kisses. And don't get me started on the intoxicating smell of her head and those beguiling eyelashes. She is rewriting our first pages of history with them.

Rationally and logically, I know these are anything but the last of our daily rituals. I don't work Fridays, and Saturday and Sunday are very much still our time and shift. Not to mention after work each and every day – and through the night, especially as the dreaded teeth descend and winter germs cast their snotty spell.

I have done this before and I rationally know that the ending of maternity service is actually the beginning of the rest of your parenting life – mixed back in with work – for better or worse. For some, it marks the first baby steps towards a reclamation of self through work and professional childcare. For others, they keep going and cannot or do not want to go back to wherever before was.

But whatever your situation when you come to this point, it doesn't stop it hurting like hell and making you feel like your insides just got all shook up. You are leaving your baby. It is hard. It is meant to be hard. For me, though, I can feel this is the right time. Although I've questioned it this week, I must admit. 'Am I going back too early?' I've asked my husband, again and again.

And yet, deep inside, I know it is the right time for me. I know I am starting to find the tidying therapeutic and then very quickly maddening and imprisoning; I am letting myself enjoy the slower pace a little too much (and the other me needs adrenaline and pace – not least to survive my pain conditions, endometriosis and adenomyosis); and my brain is idly enjoying disintegrating into loving mush.

I'm on the love slide to nothingness and everythingness and I know I need a red light in the form of an office, colleagues and a challenge beyond the octopus-armed job of mothering a baby and a five-year-old.

But knowing this and feeling this are two different things. Learning to reconcile them once more is the skill.

Retrieving my work handbag from the back of the wardrobe, stuffed with my BBC lanyard, chewed pens, a folded-up panty liner, indigestion pills and an old pack of mints, is like finding a time capsule. On the way, I pass dresses and tops from a previous me. I greet them like old friends I am getting to know again.

I can see the old me in the mirror and I tell myself I shall learn to play her again – if someone could just show me the moves and tell me the lines? I laugh ruefully. Because the old me wasn't exactly in a brilliant place, certainly not in the weeks leading up to this most recent maternity service. She was pregnant and swollen (sporting XXL Crocs in the depths of winter because no other shoes would fit) and terrified that her baby might not be safely born, as she had not long before endured a miscarriage. But then pre-pregnant me hadn't been in great shape either; stuffed full of IVF drugs and a diet of dashed hopes. *She* was in survival mode.

What I am looking for is something and someone made out of those bits but made again anew.

This doesn't stop me reaching for the same thing I did last time with our son and have done again this time with our daughter: my maternity leave letter to myself, penned as I finished my last shift at *Woman's Hour*.

I open it, a document saved on my computer, leaving the process to the last possible minute (standard practice for a hack who likes pushing her deadlines), and take a deep breath. I am in:

Dearest Emma,

This is your login and password: ******

You are good at your job and have a strong rapport with your listeners. Don't forget that.

Also don't forget you always want a big scoop but even if you don't get one for your first day, week or month back – something always happens. It always does. Always. OK?

Remember that those who matter know and those who don't, don't.

Stay off your social media mentions on Twitter and Instagram. This approach serves you well however tempting it might be to go back to peeking. I hope this maternity leave has been more of a social media detox than the last one.

Highlights before you went:

Height of nursing strikes: Pat Cullen interview
Footballer Beth Mead
Ricki Lake on her birth control doc
Kate Winslet on phones

Last show was the perfect formula: a tough minister interview, Claudia [Winkleman] and me being silly about which way to put on a loo roll and we even got TEABAGGING into the mix and a fascinating insight from the straight-talking vaccine tsar Kate Bingham.

Woman's Hour is a tapestry you weave anew every morning: ask the big question in your big hello at top.

Never do more than four items.

Let it breathe.

YOUR DAY/STRUCTURE

Night before check-in email from producer to be sent at end of their shift

Look ahead comes before debrief

Cheeky bids night before . . .

Encourage exclusives

YOU

You are still you. Somewhere in there. And even though your mind gets pulled from one tiny task to another giant one in sometimes only the space of ten seconds – you can still get into the zone. And you will do. Remember, being at home full-time isn't something that would make you happy or content – you need the contrast to be the best you can be. Plus you worked hard to get to this point of your career and just need to keep on keeping on. And if that means things are harder for a while on many levels – you need to dig in and remember this duality.

On really tough days – don't forget to properly breathe, to lower your bloody hypertonic pelvic floor and that Michelle Obama [who also had her babies via IVF] said these years of juggling small children with careers and life were tough. And she is Michelle Obama. In fact in an interview she once said:

'There were ten years where I couldn't stand my husband. And guess when it happened? When those kids were little. For ten years, while we're trying to build our careers and worrying about school and who was doing what, I was like "Argh, this isn't even." And guess what? Marriage isn't 50/50, ever.'

Channel Michelle. Because that all came pretty good.

LOVE YOU GIRL – What a show to return to xx

PS good luck and buckle the f up.

I'd also saved some messages of reassurance and luck from lovely listeners of my last *Woman's Hour*, sent before I entered the love wilderness, which I won't share here. It was all part of an attempt to fill myself with confidence, to puff my chest so I could go back with a bang.

Now as I read it all back I realize I love that I didn't know who I was writing this to: I mean, it's still the same me – but it isn't. The birth of my daughter, the child that nearly wasn't, has changed me. Again. Just like the birth of my son changed me five years earlier.

But it is also maternity service itself that rewires women – not just the having of a child. And this time, despite my best attempts, my prior knowledge and all my military-esque strategies, I was once again powerless to stop the reconfiguration. The woman writing this note nine months ago knew what she was writing but didn't fully know the woman who would be in receipt of this basic 'how to remember how to do your job' mini manual.

And yet here I am.

The letter, saved on the top right of my desktop – which has had nothing added to it in the intervening months – is still reassuring and it sends me off to my bed with a smile, like a warm chat with an old friend.

And, amazingly, I sleep. Soundly.

DAY ONE OF THE REST OF YOUR LIFE

The next morning I roll into the few clothes I know fit, laid out in preparation; silently, I brush my teeth, put on my jewellery, deodorant, make-up and perfume, and sneak out of a sleeping house like a thief stealing her identity back. Except just as I leave, my son, also an expert silent mover around a house at dawn, appears at the top of the stairs to give me the biggest kiss and to wish me luck. It is perfect timing and perfect casting. And just what I needed: the living proof that the baby I left to return to work five years ago has indeed become a human who looks forward to hearing about his mother's adventures outside of the home and away from them. I shut the door and turn on the radio in my ears, kick-starting my submersion into the wider world.

Walking back into the office does feel momentarily surreal as I see faces I haven't seen for the best part of a year as well as some brand-new ones – but I resume my old habits, and fast. I make tea for myself and my producer, brew it for four minutes while scanning my briefs, and it's reassuringly all systems go. It is helpful that a live radio programme on at ten a.m. doesn't allow for much reflection or pause. I don't think of my daughter, son or husband who will right now be navigating breakfast or pre-school reading ahead of the school run. I just work, marvelling at how the brain ramps up its speed. I swear I can almost feel the juices bubbling around my head as I restart my speed reading, send messages to people coming on to be interviewed and do some swift scriptwriting, all to the fast soundtrack of my beloved Faithless. (Somehow I have written most of my articles and scripts to the dance group's albums for the last decade. The late great Maxi Jazz and Sister Bliss's lyrics and beats soothe and inspire and are also providing this book's soundtrack too.)

Over the last three seasons as I've walked around the park with my pram-swaddled baby, I have turned over and over what my opening line on my first show back might be. I want it to be deliberately understated but tongue-in-cheek. This is finally the day I get to deliver it:

'Good morning and welcome to *Woman's Hour*. Now, where were we, then?'

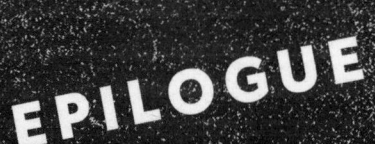
EPILOGUE

I've now been back at work for five weeks.

Once again, maternity service seems like a weird dream. I describe it in an interview as being like a land where time bends.

I see members of its population walking the streets with their prams, doing a million different tiny but important movements to comfort their small charges, but it's like I am on one side of the glass and they are on the other. I know I used to be a citizen of the same world – but I can't quite reach there again. It's a bit like pain. Despite living with it regularly, I can never quite remember how pain feels. Nor describe it. That is until I am smack bang in the middle of it again.

Despite my best efforts, my memories of maternity service continue to dim as the to-do list grows and the demands of having two jobs, office and home, and a need for some kind of selfish fun SOMEWHERE in the mix, dominate.

While the rhythm of work has settled within and around me more and more, the tiredness has yet to abate. As has the feeling of not quite managing to toggle between the two countries, the two selves.

Now I am split. And even though I've done it before, I am struggling to remember the dance moves. The switch between work me and home me isn't smooth yet. It's jagged and harsh; a work in progress not particularly aided by broken nights.

Unbelievably, I find myself missing the purity of maternity service – the single-mindedness of it and the aimless pottering. The focus on what was important as opposed to transient work decisions and dramas. And even though my mind was deadened, it was at least 100 per cent where it had to be. The rose-tinted glasses are firmly clamped back on to my tired face as I am no longer interested in faithfully remembering how it actually felt. Screw accuracy. I am all mush.

The two handbags on the armchair in the hallway start to take on a greater significance: a physical manifestation of my two selves. The smaller one contains my work pass, headphones, two lipsticks, a news magazine, blusher and a full wallet. The other? Lego, nappies, wipes, tissues, bum cream, soft toys, lip balm and two hair bobbles. And a range of hats and muslins.

Which one is me? Both. And then some.

The romanticizing and rewriting of my maternity service as a dreamy existence is given a short, sharp and messy reality check when my daughter takes an almighty poo in the bath. Unprepared, I scrabble about trying to figure out what to do with her and with my naked five-year-old who is preparing to jump into what is now a sewer. I realize that, post my work shift, I had been briefly lulled out of the state of parental hypervigilance. I had only been thinking of her chubby cheeks and all her delicious softness; the divine way she now claps when she sees me and pats my face. I had forgotten about her less than delicious habits.

An older work friend drily texts later after I check in: *Emma, that's why I always kept a sieve in the bathroom.* I laugh and then lack the energy to retort that we aren't that solid yet but thanks for the tip. More fibre is definitely needed.

That's when it dawns on me: I had been expecting to feel pleasure at my return to work, at what I had thought would be my return to self. And while there has been satisfaction, the reality is that work isn't a holiday away from home. Neither is home a chilled-out zone. What I am craving is a break, not *more* work. The old kind of break you used to get after work and before children. The freedom to simply be, and the fulfilment of the desire to be alone. Or to go properly wild without thinking of responsibilities back at base. And *then* return to your family. Now I understand that this is the part of returning to work that doesn't really return.

Going back to work has given me back some sanity, my sense of self and a much-needed financial boost – but there are some post-maternity-service yearnings it doesn't fulfil. If anything, being back at work has made it harder to seize those opportunities when I feel I need to occasionally just be *me* – so desperate am I to see my children in the allotted hours we have together.

Even on your best day at work, you don't go there for the release and fun of it. Even on your best homecoming to very small children, after a long working week, you don't go there for the release and fun of it.

Yet there *is* fun to be found in both scenarios, and in

the latter I have experienced some of the warmest feelings of contentment I have ever known (often when I least expected them).

As I settle back into this toggling between work and caring for two very young children, I have come to realize it is my maternity service that has given me the tools I can deploy right now to try and feel satisfaction in both parts of my life: a sense of duty and a sense of service. During those months in the trenches I discovered that when you dig in hardest – even, and especially, when you feel like you can't be bothered – you always end up feeling better. (It's a bit like going to the gym.)

At home when I do something to truly help my children, or something thoughtful that makes their world a bit brighter, it gives me such a sense of happiness and satisfaction. Like reading to our son and washing his comforter in time for bed, still warm from the dryer. He is thrilled and so I am – it's just a very different kind of thrill to the thrills I experienced before having children.

Similarly at work, when I prioritize making a tray of teas for the studio team, just before we go live, while finishing writing the last part of the scripts, I realize I now have more perspective about how we need to feel before the show starts, as well as the product being ready. Somehow through the course of my maternity service I have learned to create more time within the same time window (and massively prioritize hot drinks).

The sense of duty I learned on maternity service, flavoured with the deepest love I have ever known, is the secret sauce that just about keeps this show on the road.

That and a wee dram. Preferably neat.

Reassuringly, the broadcaster Dame Joan Bakewell recently described her small-children-rearing years as passing in 'duty and indulgence'. She also confessed to hating it and getting bored, because she wasn't working during that period. Despite being ninety-one, she remembers these feelings very clearly and yet still gets on very well with both her daughter and son. But there's that word again: *duty*.

It has been there all along. And I forget it at my peril.

FOREWARNED
IS FOREARMED

As I said back at the beginning of this book, I have written this in order to remember, and for my daughter to be forearmed and prepared. I want you and your daughters to be armed too.

So, here are some final tactics:

- Think of maternity leave as maternity *service*.
- Duty, service, sacrifice, routine, uniform, recovery, love: rinse and repeat.
- Go in with your eyes and heart open. It's wild and it will take you to brinks and edges of yourself you may never see again.
- You won't remember most of it, neither the smells nor the sheer repetitiveness of the tasks. Nor will your baby.
- But you will remember some – and rightly the best parts: the first smile, giggle, baby tooth, rollover, eye contact and words.
- You will remember what your baby was like, but not how it was for you at this time. Again – a clever part of humanity's design.
- This period of your life is finite and you will get there – wherever there is.

- Anyone who knows, knows. Even if they don't say it. Or feel it entirely.
- Your child is incredible and so are you.
- Maternity service is extraordinary, exhausting, frustrating, mind-altering, bewildering, enraging, heart-opening. And, amazingly, forgettable. Forgetting it, though, does a major disservice – to the women who came before us (without any domestic appliances) and the women who are to come.

So, thank you for your service.

If you can, pass this on.

And please never, ever forget.